# Fck Menorrhagia

# Contents

# Welcome to the Flood Zone

If you've ever stood up and felt something ominous shift—like the soundtrack to a horror movie cueing up—you're part of an elite, unspoken sisterhood. The ones who don't just "get their period." That's amateur hour. This is something else entirely. This is **menorrhagia**—aka Shark Week on steroids, aka The Red Wedding, aka "Did I just pass out, or did my jeans just die?"

This book isn't for the faint of heart or the light of flow. If you're one of those mythical creatures who chirp, *"I barely notice my period!"*—congratulations, Barbie. Go rollerblade in white pants. The rest of us? We're crime-scene custodians of our own bedsheets. We're warriors strapping on heating pads like chest armor. We're tampon-layering engineers, building blood barriers with every overpriced product on the pharmacy shelf.

Menorrhagia isn't "a little extra." It's a condition that sounds like it was named after a Roman goddess of vengeance—and she's coming for your energy, your paycheck, your social calendar, and your mat-

# Contents

# Welcome to the Flood Zone

If you've ever stood up and felt something ominous shift—like the soundtrack to a horror movie cueing up—you're part of an elite, unspoken sisterhood. The ones who don't just "get their period." That's amateur hour. This is something else entirely. This is **menorrhagia**—aka Shark Week on steroids, aka The Red Wedding, aka "Did I just pass out, or did my jeans just die?"

This book isn't for the faint of heart or the light of flow. If you're one of those mythical creatures who chirp, *"I barely notice my period!"*—congratulations, Barbie. Go rollerblade in white pants. The rest of us? We're crime-scene custodians of our own bedsheets. We're warriors strapping on heating pads like chest armor. We're tampon-layering engineers, building blood barriers with every overpriced product on the pharmacy shelf.

Menorrhagia isn't "a little extra." It's a condition that sounds like it was named after a Roman goddess of vengeance—and she's coming for your energy, your paycheck, your social calendar, and your mattress. It's soaking through in thirty minutes. It's canceling work because you bled through your coat. It's telling a doctor, *"I'm losing too much blood,"* and getting handed iron pills like that's gonna plug the Red Sea.

And the worst part? Nobody cares.

The world coos that periods are "natural" and "beautiful." Sure, maybe if you're not bleeding like a gutted deer on a three-week schedule. But for us? It's praying in a public restroom that your backup pad didn't shift like tectonic plates. It's running out of outfits halfway through vacation. It's being told to "tough it out" while wondering if you should head to the ER or start writing your will.

So, let's talk about it. Let's roast it. Let's drag the ignorance, the gaslighting, the "just drink tea" advice, and the sorry excuse for products we've been force-fed since middle school.

This is not the cute self-care guide with pastel infographics and affirmations. This is the brutally honest, sarcastic, medically accurate, darkly hilarious manual you wish someone handed you the first time you bled through a hotel towel and smuggled it home in your suitcase like contraband.

Welcome to the Flood Zone. Welcome to the Red Wedding. We're not being quiet anymore.

# 1

# The Moment You Stand Up

There's a specific moment that anyone with menorrhagia knows too well. It's not when the cramps start. Not even when the bloating kicks in. No, it's that cursed moment when you stand up after sitting for a while—and feel your uterus empty itself like a dam breaking in biblical times.

You freeze. You clench. You pray to the tampon gods, the pad gods, the cotton blend gods. You shuffle to the nearest restroom like a penguin trying not to disturb an explosive device strapped to their underwear. You hope. You pray. You check.

And it's never good.

You see, regular period-havers don't understand this hell. They can cough. They can laugh. They can run. They live like carefree tampon models doing backflips in commercials. You, on the other hand, have to approach life like you're transporting unstable plutonium in your pants.

Let's not sugarcoat this: menorrhagia is *not* a heavy period. It's a damn blood sacrifice. It's bleeding through two pads and a super tampon in less than an hour. It's ruining every pair of jeans you ever loved. It's wearing black leggings year-round like a goth ninja—not because you're edgy, but because you don't trust your uterus to behave in public.

And God help you if you're not home when it happens.

**Let's Paint a Bloody Picture**

You're in a meeting. Or church. Or your friend's wedding. You've been sitting for 45 minutes. Things feel... manageable. But then you stand up—and there it is. That warm, unmistakable rush. You don't even have to look. You know. It's happening. You are leaking like a sink pipe that's been duct-taped shut by lies.

You grab your purse like a CIA agent on a mission, nodding fake smiles as you excuse yourself. You're not okay. You are one sneeze away from a crimson crime scene.

In the bathroom, you inspect the damage. It's bad. Your pad gave up. Your tampon waved the white flag. Your underwear looks like it lost a turf war. And if you didn't bring backup? Sis, you're straight up *screwed.*

## Let's Talk Logistics

This condition forces you to become a logistics queen. You plan outfits like you're prepping for a blood-heavy battlefield. Want to wear white? Are you high? Want to sit on a friend's beige couch? Not unless you hate them. You don't leave the house without pads, wipes, underwear, Advil, and the jaded, thousand-yard stare of someone who's seen too much.

You learn how to track your flow like a storm chaser. You know your bathroom access points in every building. You've scoped out restrooms in grocery stores, gas stations, public parks—hell, you've probably MacGyvered makeshift pads from toilet paper and despair more times than you can count.

And then there's the dreaded car seat moment. That white-knuckled second when you stand up from your car and glance back like you're checking for bodies. You don't want to see it—but you have to look. If your seat survived, you praise God. If it didn't? You wrap a hoodie around your waist and drive straight to your shame spiral.

## The Sleep Setup That Deserves an Engineering Degree

Sleep is no longer rest. It's risk.

You don't just lie down like a normal person. You build a perimeter: towel, old sheets, waterproof pad, backup towel, heating pad, maybe a sacrificial shirt from an ex you never liked anyway. You sleep like a hostage in your own bed, barely moving, because if you roll over too fast, it's game over.

And even with all that prep? You still wake up to a mess. You strip the bed like it's a crime scene and hope you can salvage the mattress without leaving a giant shame stamp on it. And if you're staying over at someone else's place? May God have mercy on your soul. There's no panic like the 6 a.m. sneak-clean operation trying to scrub blood out of someone's guest sheets with hand soap and tears.

## And Don't Even Get Me Started on Public Embarrassment

Let's talk about *that* moment. You know the one.

You're walking through Target, living your best life. Suddenly someone taps your shoulder. "Hey... I think you have something on the back of your pants."

No.

You didn't feel it happen. It betrayed you silently. Your uterus is shady like that—striking when you're distracted by snacks or seasonal clearance aisles.

4

You speed-walk to the restroom, check the mirror, and yep. You look like you sat in ketchup. Only it ain't ketchup. And now you gotta find a hoodie, tie it around your waist, and do the walk of menstrual shame to your car like you're fleeing a massacre.

You sit in the car and contemplate your entire existence. You wonder why no one cares. You wonder if any other condition would be treated with this much casual neglect.

If men had this problem, there'd be a federal Menorrhagia Relief Act with free Uber rides, dedicated clot-busting tech, and monthly care packages hand-delivered by trained professionals.

**The Emotional Toll Nobody Talks About**

Let's be real. Menorrhagia isn't just physical. It's mental warfare.

You live in a state of anxiety. You dread leaving the house. You cancel plans. You don't feel sexy. You don't feel in control. You feel like a prisoner of your own body. You feel like something's wrong, but every doctor says it's "normal." Spoiler: It's not.

You cry. You rage. You want to throw your uterus into the ocean and wish it luck. You start Googling hysterectomies and end up spiraling through horror stories. You drink tea. You try acupuncture. You pray. You bleed. Rinse and repeat.

You start hiding it. You make jokes. You shrug it

off. You smile while sitting on a literal heating pad in a Zoom call. And everyone assumes you're fine.

You are not fine. You are a survivor. Every damn month.

## This Chapter Is for the Ones Who Thought It Was Just Them

Let me make this loud and clear: if you've ever felt insane for bleeding so much… you're not. If you've ever walked out of a gynecologist's office feeling dismissed or gaslit… you're not crazy. If you've ever bled through your clothes and still had to smile through a work shift… you are a goddamn warrior.

This condition is real. It's under-researched. It's under-discussed. And it's massively under-treated. It can destroy your iron levels, ruin your energy, wreck your confidence, and still get brushed off as "just part of being a woman."

This book is not here to coddle. It's here to call sh*t out.

Because while the world keeps making blue-liquid pad commercials with acrobatic dancers, we're out here bleaching sheets and canceling dates because we literally can't stop bleeding long enough to feel like humans.

## And If You're Reading This While Sitting on a

**Towel...**

You're not alone.

You might be leaking through your third pad in an hour. You might be clenching your thighs together in public. You might be one exhale away from a disaster.

But you're also a walking miracle.

You've dealt with this for years and you're still standing. Still working. Still surviving. You deserve answers. You deserve options. You deserve a mattress that isn't a war zone.

And if no one else is gonna say it? Then let this be the moment you hear it loud:

*F*ck menorrhagia.*

# 2

# Super Plus? Sis, I Need the HAZMAT Version

Let's go ahead and address the big cotton lie we've all been fed: that somewhere out there exists a magical product capable of taming the beast known as menorrhagia.

Lies. All lies.

There is no pad. No tampon. No "super plus ultra mega" hybrid. No unicorn-certified menstrual cup infused with monk tears. This is beyond regular period gear. This is **emergency preparedness.**

Menorrhagia warriors don't *shop* for protection. We **stockpile** it. FEMA should be issuing us gear. NASA should be consulting us on fluid containment. Instead, we're crouched in pharmacy aisles decoding absorbency charts like they're rocket launch instructions.

*Tampons: The Great Letdown*

That box that says *"Super Plus"*? Cute.

Insert one, blink twice, and boom—it's soaked like it belly-flopped into a swimming pool. Those "8 hours of protection" printed on the box? More like 45 minutes, and that's if you sit perfectly still. Add movement, coughing, or God forbid, laughter—and you're one sneeze away from disaster.

And those organic tampons? Lovely for people with polite, whisper-light periods. But if your uterus is reenacting a medieval battle, the eco-friendly vibes won't save your jeans.

*Pads: The Adult Diaper Struggle*

Pads are supposed to be the barrier between your blood tsunami and the rest of society. You'd think they'd be engineered like tanks. Instead, we get "wings."

Ma'am, I don't need my pad to fly. I need it to **stay put** during a full-scale bleed-out.

And those "overnight" pads claiming 12 hours of protection? Maybe for ghosts. By hour two you're walking like you're smuggling a soggy tortilla in your pants.

## The Menstrual Cup Myth

Ah, the menstrual cup: the minimalist's dream, the eco-warrior's badge of honor. Until you try removing it mid-flood.

Breaking that seal during a menorrhagia surge is like emptying a fish tank with a shot glass. One slip, and it's *Carrie (1976)* in your bathroom—blood on your hands, legs, and floor. Drop the cup in the toilet? Congratulations, you've just unlocked the bonus round of Hell.

If cups work for you, amazing. Truly. But please don't stroll in here saying *"just try it!"* like it's a Pinterest hack. Some of us are surviving a biblical flood, not hosting a craft fair.

## The Double-Up Hustle

Tampon first. Then pad. Maybe two pads. Some even add a pantyliner horizontally across the back like a seatbelt. That's the level of innovation happening here.

Bathroom trips become tactical operations: check, shift, replace, reinforce. Forget thongs. We wear **Period Armor**™—high-rise, full-coverage underwear that could double as parachutes in an emergency.

*The Lies We Were Told in School*

Remember that middle school "health talk"? Some awkward lady pulled out a pad the size of a bookmark and whispered, *"This should last a few hours."*
  Ma'am. That barely lasts through a sneeze.
  We were set up. We should've had **drills**:

- "Here's how to change a tampon in a moving car without flashing truckers."
- "Here's how to unstick a menstrual cup in a gas station bathroom without crying."
- "Here's how to exit a date gracefully when your uterus reenacts the Red Sea."

*Emergency Bleed Kits Should Be Real*

Forget cute makeup bags. We need FEMA-style go-bags stocked with:

- Heavy-duty tampons
- Ultra-thick pads
- Black leggings
- Ibuprofen
- Hydration powder
- Chocolate
- A full change of underwear
- A mattress topper

- And, honestly, a murder alibi

Because this isn't "a cycle." This is a **rupture.** If a regular period is a faucet, menorrhagia is a busted fire hydrant in July.

*The "It Can't Be That Bad" Crowd*

Here's the kicker: people who don't have menorrhagia always doubt us.

"Oh come on, it's just your period."

No. It's a medical condition.

"You're exaggerating."

Really? Then why am I iron deficient every month like a character in a Victorian novel? Why am I losing blood at levels that qualify me to star in a vampire documentary?

The worst part is you start to doubt yourself. But hear me: you're not crazy. The products suck. The system sucks. *You do not.*

*How About Real Solutions?*

Yes, treatments exist—hormonal therapy, ablation, IUDs, surgery. But getting them? Like auditioning for *American Idol.*

- Track your cycle like a NASA analyst.

- Prove you've bled through every Target outfit in stock.
- Beg your doctor.
- Argue why you're not "being dramatic" while your hemoglobin's on life support.

And even then, many of us just get iron pills tossed our way with a *"Let's wait and see."* Wait and see what—if I pass out in Costco?

*We Deserve Better. Period.*

This isn't glitter. This isn't exaggeration. It's blood. Treat it accordingly.

We deserve products that work for us, not just for yoga influencers with polite, four-day fairy flows. We deserve science, funding, innovation, and—bare minimum—warning labels that stop pretending tampons last eight hours.

Menorrhagia is not "just a period." It's survival. And survival deserves respect.

# 3

# Your Bed Is a Crime Scene

There's no preparing for it. No matter how many towels, mattress pads, or "period-safe" sheets you stack, when menorrhagia hits at night your bed becomes a war zone. And not just any war—this is medieval battlefield energy.

You wake up groggy. Something feels wrong. Damp. Sticky. Betrayal. You sit up slowly, terrified to look. But you know. Another set of sheets gone. Another towel failed. The pad-and-tampon tag team? Both tapped out hours ago. You shuffle to the bathroom like you're starring in a low-budget slasher flick.

There's blood on your thighs. On your legs. Somehow on your pillow. You mutter curses like an exorcist while stripping the bed. You pour peroxide like holy water. You Google "how to get blood out of memory foam" for the fiftieth time. And even when it looks clean, you know. Deep in the mattress. Deep in your soul. You know.

And the worst part? This isn't a freak accident. This is monthly. This is your life.

*The Bedtime Ritual*

Insomniacs think they have it bad? Try sleeping with a uterus that betrays you nightly. You don't "go to bed." You build a fortress:

1. Towel (already bleach-stained)
2. Mattress protector (retired years ago)
3. Waterproof pad (slips the moment you exhale)
4. Sacrificial comforter
5. Period underwear stacked like lasagna
6. Lie frozen in one position till morning

Every hour, your inner voice whispers: *"Check your ass. You're leaking."*

*Sharing a Bed: A Trust Fall From Hell*

Husband, hookup, dog—it doesn't matter. Anyone sharing your bed is either on the cleanup crew or about to be traumatized.

You warn them:

*"Listen, it's like a biblical plague every month."*

They laugh. They think you're exaggerating. Then 6 a.m. hits and they wake up looking like they starred in *Saw IV: Uterus Edition.*

If they're cool, they grab towels. If not, you'll find them ranting on Reddit about "a woman who ruined my 800-thread count sheets."

*Mattress PTSD*

Eventually you stop shopping for pretty bedding. You shop for camouflage.

- White? Forbidden.
- Beige? Too risky.
- Pastels? Only if you hate yourself.
- Black or burgundy? The new neutral.

At some point you stop buying new sheets altogether. Why bother? You know what's coming. Even your mattress groans when you lie down—it's seen too much.

*Travel Panic*

Hotels and Airbnbs? A nightmare.

You pack towels, old pillowcases, a whole survival kit. You armor up and still wake up to betrayal. Cue the covert ops:

- Scrubbing sheets with hotel soap
- Blow-drying stains at 5 a.m.
- Flipping mattresses like you're hiding a body

You've never committed a crime, but you've covered up enough evidence to be indicted.

*Talking to Bedding Like It's Alive*

You've said it:
  "Come on, towel. Hold the line."
  "Be strong, sheet. You got this."
  "RIP fitted sheet, she fought bravely."
  It's half joke, half prayer. You're one leak away from a breakdown.

*Clots: The Unspoken Horror*

Nobody prepared us for the clots. You wake up, stagger to the bathroom, and pass something that feels like you birthed a jellyfish. You stare at the toilet like, *"Should I call a priest?"*

And somehow, you're expected to rinse your hands, grab a coffee, and head to work.

## The Morning Damage Report

Every morning is CSI: Uterus Edition. You inspect the sheets. The leggings. The mattress. The underwear. Half survived, half didn't. You sigh, hands on hips, and whisper, *"How am I still alive?"*

Then you grab the bleach. Again.

## Let's Be Clear

This isn't "just a period." This is a recurring, body-wrecking condition. Losing sleep. Ruining property. Bleeding out chunks that could qualify as evidence. And we're told to "tough it out"? No.

## Final Thoughts: Respect the Survivors

We hold jobs. We raise kids. We maintain relationships. All while secretly fearing our beds will betray us again tonight.

So when someone laughs about periods, tell them this:

*"My mattress has seen things. Things that would make Netflix cancel itself out of pity."*

# 4

# Doctors Who Gaslight You Into Insanity

Going to the doctor for menorrhagia feels less like getting care and more like standing trial. You're bleeding like a slow-motion horror film, laying out the evidence: *"I wake up in blood. I bleed through a super plus tampon in 30 minutes. My life is scheduled around bathrooms."*

And what do you get?

A smile.

A "hmm."

The infamous head tilt.

Followed by: *"Well, everyone's flow is different."*

Cue the internal scream.

*Welcome to the Gaslight Games*

You describe the ruined clothes. The ruined bed. The constant exhaustion. You say the words, *"I'm scared I'll bleed out in my sleep."*

Their answer? *"Have you tried birth control?"*

That's it. The big reveal. As if a pack of pills is going to dam the Red Sea. Already on birth control? Then it must not be "that bad."

Excuse me? Tell that to my mattress.


*The Hemoglobin Hustle*

Even when your labs scream *"anemia"*—dizzy, pale, hemoglobin on E—they still shift blame.

"You need more iron in your diet."

Ma'am, I could lick a cast-iron skillet and still end up deficient. Because no amount of spinach fixes a sword wound happening monthly.


*The Stress Shuffle*

Complain about pain, and suddenly you're not hemorrhaging—you're "stressed."

You could walk in holding a bucket of your own blood and the doctor would still ask, *"Have you tried mindfulness?"*

Translation: "You're dramatic."

*When Male Doctors Chime In*

The only thing worse than dismissal is condescension.

You explain *flooding.*

He smiles knowingly: *"My wife has heavy periods, too."*

Sir. That's not a credential. That's a red flag. Unless you've bled through denim at brunch, keep your wife out of my chart.


*OB-GYN Roulette*

Finding a good doctor is like spinning a wheel: compassionate specialist… or human shrug in scrubs.

Best case: they run real tests.

Worst case: they drop gems like *"Periods are supposed to be inconvenient."*

Oh really? So is open-heart surgery, but y'all don't tell patients to "tough it out."


*The Appointment Script*

- You: *"I've been bleeding heavily for years, I'm exhausted, I think I'm dying."*
- Doctor: *"Are you sexually active?"*
- You: *"Yes, but I'm here about my period."*
- Doctor: *"Could you be pregnant?"*

- You: *"...Not unless I conceived by osmosis."*
- Doctor: *"Hmm. Let's try the pill."*

And out you go—more confused, more broke, and still bleeding.

## *Testing Delays*

Want an ultrasound? Beg. Want a hysteroscopy? Six referrals. By the time you get a real diagnosis, you've bled through half your closet and developed medical trauma worthy of its own memoir.

Then comes the kicker: *"Why didn't you come in sooner?"*

Because I did. For years. Y'all said "it's hormones" and sent me home with Flintstones vitamins.

## *Birth Control Isn't a Magic Wand*

Birth control is the universal prescription for everything: acne, cramps, hemorrhaging like a Civil War reenactment.

When it doesn't work—or makes you worse—it's never the treatment, always you. *"You didn't take it right. Try another brand. Give it more time."*

Meanwhile you're on your fifth pill, cycling between nonstop bleeding, mood spirals, and bloating like a balloon animal. But sure—let's spin the roulette wheel again.

*The Guilt Game*

On top of dismissal, you get scolded:
    "You're not compliant."
    "You're anxious."
    "You just need to adjust."
    Translation: *"We don't have answers, so we'll blame you instead."*
    You came in for help. You leave feeling like you failed a test you never signed up for.

*What You Deserve Instead*

If you're waking up in blood, passing clots that look like special-effects props, and dragging yourself through life, you deserve an **investigation**, not excuses. Full hormone panels. Imaging. Iron monitoring. A treatment plan that isn't just, "Here, swallow this and shut up."

*If Men Had Menorrhagia...*

There'd be grants. Campaigns. Apps. Netflix specials titled *Bleeding Out: The Men's Crisis.* Entire startups dedicated to clot-catching underwear. Emergency leave policies. And a Menorrhagia Relief

Act signed into law yesterday.

But because it's women? It's "just a period."

*Final Mic-Drop*

This isn't drama. This isn't a quirky inconvenience. This is pathology—chronic, brutal, and life-wrecking.

So next time a doctor tilts their head and says, *"Everyone's flow is different,"* you have every right to look them in the eye and reply:

*"And everyone's bullshit tolerance is different. Mine just ran out."*

Because you're not crazy. You're not "just hormonal." You're bleeding out and still showing up. That makes you a warrior. And if doctors won't take your bleeding seriously, just wait until you try explaining it to a guy on a first date.

# 5

## Dating While Hemorrhaging Like a Stab Victim

Dating with menorrhagia is a biohazard romance adventure. Every potential night out has a risk factor somewhere between *"light dinner"* and *"oops, I left a trail."*

And before anyone suggests "just plan dates around your cycle," let me stop you right there.

What cycle?

With menorrhagia, your period shows up early, stays late, drops in twice a month, or lurks with random spotting like it forgot its keys. There's no planning. Just chaos. And somehow, you're supposed to date through that?

*The First Date Outfit: NASA Edition*

You want to look hot. You also don't want to ruin restaurant seating. So you assemble the survival fit:

- Black pants, always.
- Loose top, because bloat.
- Period underwear under another layer of black panties.
- Tampon + pad combo.
- Backup underwear, leggings, and wipes in your purse.
- Hoodie to tie around your waist if betrayal strikes.

You don't walk out the door cute—you walk out tactical. Sexy Navy SEAL, mission: don't bleed in public.

*The Hug Hazard*

He leans in for a hug. You freeze.

Not because you're shy, but because you just felt a clot shift and your tampon might have clocked out. You side-hug like an aunt at Thanksgiving. He looks puzzled. You're just trying not to christen his shirt.

## Bathroom Recon

The most important part of date-night strategy? Bathrooms.

You need a restaurant with clean stalls, close to the table, preferably single-occupancy because you're about to do covert menstruation surgery in there.

You excuse yourself like, *"Powdering my nose!"* but inside it's advanced origami: tampon swap, pad shift, wipe down, inspection, whisper a pep talk to your uterus, and exit like nothing happened. Lip gloss check for cover.

## The Gravity Betrayal

Sit too long and it pools. Stand up and—bam—gravity plays "Release the Kraken."

You clench, shuffle, and speed-walk to the restroom like you're hiding contraband, praying your backup system held. Meanwhile, your date wonders why you vanish every 40 minutes like a menstruating Carmen Sandiego.

## The Couch Dilemma

Date's going well? He invites you back? Cute. But your brain immediately asks:

- "What color is the couch?"
- "What if I sneeze?"
- "Do I sit on a hoodie like a puppy pad?"

You smile, nod, accept—but never relax. Every cuddle is just another opportunity for betrayal.

*To Tell or Not to Tell*

Do you casually drop, *"Hey, I bleed like a horror set once a month and it's happening right now"*?

Didn't think so.

You joke about being "a geyser," they laugh politely, but nobody really gets it. They nod like they're ready, but nothing prepares someone for dinner followed by *Gladiator: Uterus Edition.*

*Sex: Logistics, Not Lust*

If you're down for period intimacy, with menorrhagia it's not sex—it's an engineering project.

- Towels.
- Painkillers.
- Low lighting.
- A cleanup plan that rivals CSI.

Half the time you just cancel. You say you're tired,

"not in the mood," or "laying low." Really? You're protecting them from witnessing a scene that could traumatize a crime lab intern.

*The Emotional Toll*

Here's the part people don't talk about: the shame.

Feeling like you're "too much." Feeling like you need to apologize for bleeding. Feeling undateable because your body refuses to be chill.

It eats at you. But the truth? You're not the problem. Your uterus is just a diva who won't clock out.

*Meanwhile, Men*

Men stroll into dates carefree, dry, in white shorts, with nothing to worry about except ordering appetizers. Must be nice.

You, meanwhile, are defusing tampon bombs in an Applebee's bathroom.

*Why You're Still Winning*

And yet—you still show up. You still flirt. You still crack jokes. You still look good. You still carry conversations while leaking like a faucet.

Anybody can date when they feel perfect. But

showing up mid-hemorrhage? That's bad bitch energy. That's resilience. That's elite-level functioning under pressure.

*The Real Test*

If someone can't handle that you menstruate like a chainsaw massacre, they don't deserve you. You need someone who:

- Doesn't flinch at the word "clot."
- Hands you a heating pad without asking.
- Doesn't blink when you say, "Bathroom again!"
- Treats you like a person, not a problem.

*Final Word*

Dating with menorrhagia isn't weakness—it's endurance. You've bled through jeans, slept on towels, MacGyvered pads in moving cars, and you're still here, lip gloss on, cracking jokes across the table.

So if someone asks what makes you strong, you can tell them:

*"I survived this date while hemorrhaging. What have you survived lately?"*

Mic drop. Napkin dab. Smile. Carry on.

# 6

# The Cost of Bleeding for a Living

You ever look at your bank account and realize most of your money literally went down the drain? Welcome to the glamorous, overpriced hellscape of bleeding too much in a world that still calls it "just a minor inconvenience."

This chapter is for every girl who had to choose between gas or tampons. For everyone who's dropped $80 in a month on pads, pain meds, leggings, and new sheets. For every soul who walked into CVS for Midol and left with a receipt long enough to double as gauze.

This isn't just a health issue. It's a financial hostage situation.

*The Real Numbers*

They say the "average woman" spends about $13 a month on period products. That's cute.

Now here's the heavy-flow starter pack:

- Super-plus tampons (2 boxes): $18
- Overnight pads (2 packs): $16
- Painkillers: $10
- Period underwear: $30+ a pair
- Black leggings (after another casualty): $20
- Mattress protector (again): $30
- Iron supplements: $12
- Heating pad replacement: $25
- Laundry detergent & stain remover: $10+
- Chocolate (mandatory): $6

**Grand total:** $165–200 a month.

And that's if you don't end up in the ER.


*Insurance? You Thought.*

Trying to get insurance to cover menorrhagia is like asking your landlord to fix the heat this year.

Tests? Hundreds.

Ultrasounds? More hundreds.

Specialist? $180 for a five-minute chat ending with *"Try birth control."*

And if you push harder? Suddenly it's all "elective." Elective? As if you chose to Jackson Pollock your sheets every three weeks.

*The Blood Budget*

A typical week looks like this:

- Day 1: Tampons, pads, Advil = $45
- Day 2: Ruined underwear = $18
- Day 3: Emergency leggings = $25
- Day 4: Missed work = $120 lost wages
- Day 5: Supplies ran out = $30
- Day 6: DoorDash binge because cramps = $50
- Day 7: Still bleeding = priceless

And society shrugs: *"Periods are natural!"*

So are earthquakes. Doesn't mean we shouldn't do something about them.

*Work Doesn't Care*

Try calling in:

*"Hey boss, I can't come in. I'm bleeding like a gutted deer."*

*"Sorry, that's not a valid reason."*

If this much blood came from a nose, you'd be admitted to the ER. But because it's uterine, you're expected to power through, fake a smile, and hope your pad holds through the morning meeting.

No PTO for clots. No HR sympathy for fainting at your register. Just "grind harder."

*Period Poverty: Menorrhagia Edition*

People frame "period poverty" as something far away. But it's happening in your apartment.

You're out here calculating whether to double up pads or rewear stained jeans so you can afford rent. You're replacing underwear, towels, even mattresses while someone tells you $13 a month should cover it.

This isn't period poverty. This is menorrhagia bankruptcy.

*The Luxury Scam*

Why are pads wrapped like high-end chocolates? Why are tampons marketed like spa products?

I don't need butterflies on a box. I need flood control. They brag about "overnight protection" like it's a hotel mattress. Sis, I'm not sleeping. I'm in battle.

## Why Isn't This Free Yet?

If men bled once a month, tampons would be stacked free next to ketchup packets. Pads would be tax-deductible. Every bathroom would have dispensers, heating pads, and a nurse on standby.

But because it's women, we get a pastel box with flowers on it and a surcharge for existing.

## The Hidden Taxes

The bleeding bill doesn't stop at products. Add in:

- Replacing clothes, towels, bedding
- Extra laundry loads
- Cancelled social events = emotional tax
- Missed workouts = health tax
- Takeout comfort food = survival tax
- Upgrading hotel rooms for private bathrooms

Every month is a fresh invoice your uterus sends straight to your wallet.

## And Yet You Still Show Up

You still work. Cook. Parent. Pay bills. Smile in public while hemorrhaging like your uterus is breaking out of prison.

You bleed for free while being told it's no big deal. That isn't just strength—it's unpaid labor. And the world should be ashamed for expecting it.

*Final Tally*

You pay to hide your pain. You pay to make others comfortable. You pay to keep going while your body betrays you.

But let's call it what it is: bullshit.

You deserve more access, more resources, more empathy, more options. Free products. Real coverage. Real care.

Until then, the invoice is clear:

*Fck the tampon tax. F*ck the gaslighting. And f*ck the idea that your suffering is "just part of being a woman." But money isn't the only thing bleeding us dry — society has its own way of pretending this isn't a big deal.

# 7

# Society Pretending It's Not That Bad

Ah yes, society. The same civilization that built drones, AI, and self-warming coffee mugs… but still acts like women hemorrhaging monthly is either taboo or comedy material.

Welcome to the gaslit Hunger Games, where your uterus is staging a coup and the world's response is: *"Have you tried yoga?"*

## Media: The Blue Liquid Lie

Commercials show a smiling woman in white pants, horseback riding, jogging, fist-bumping friends, while neat blue Windex pours onto a pad.

Reality? You hunched over a space heater, swallowing ibuprofen like Tic Tacs, praying your pad holds another hour.

But advertisers insist periods are dainty whispers.

Never the full-body hemorrhage they actually are.

*Workplaces: Bleed in Silence*

Try asking for time off because you're hemorrhaging.

Boss: *"We're short-staffed."*

Coworker: *"Take a Tylenol."*

Imagine a man gushing blood from his nose for seven days, fainting mid-meeting. He'd be rushed to the ER. You? You're expected to smile and finish the PowerPoint. Mention your period and suddenly you're "oversharing."

*Public Bathrooms: Torture Chambers*

Ever change a tampon in a stall designed by someone who's clearly never had a uterus?

No hooks. No shelves. Auto-flush spraying your ass mid-change. Trash cans stationed 12 feet away, forcing you to Kobe a blood-soaked pad across the room. Sometimes there's no trash can at all—because apparently we just... don't bleed.

*Period Leave? In This Economy?*

Japan and parts of Europe have it. Here? You're lucky if HR doesn't label you "emotional" for missing a day.

Explain to a male manager: *"I feel like I might faint from blood loss, but I'll try to push through."*

Him: *"Cool, but can you send that report first?"*


*Health Class Lies*

They told us: "3–7 days."

They told us: "A little discomfort."

They handed us a pamphlet and a free pad.

Meanwhile, real life is 10-day hemorrhages, clot-passing horror shows, and jeans ruined in the Target aisle. Education failed us before we even started.


*The Red Silence*

Men can watch guts spill on TV. But talk about your actual blood loss in real life? "Too graphic."

Movies: Explosions, disembowelment, carnage.

You: "I passed a clot."

Them: *"Whoa, TMI."*

The hypocrisy is louder than your heating pad.

*Period Shame: The Hidden Tax*

You've:

- Cried hiding a leak.
- Apologized for bleeding.
- Wrapped a sweater around your waist like a spy cover.
- Whispered "check my butt" like it's code.

That's shame, drilled into us so deep we don't even question it. Society made us think our bodies are gross for doing what they do.

*Speak Up, Get Mocked*

Tweet about your pain? Trolls.
   Push for healthcare? "It's not that serious."
   Tell your doctor? *"My girlfriend doesn't complain."*
   She probably does—just not to you, Chad.

*The Casualness of Misery*

We joke to survive:
   *"Oh, I bled through my third pair of jeans."*
   *"Oh, I passed a clot the size of a chicken nugget."*
   If men endured that, there'd be an annual medical summit named after it. For us? It's "just Tuesday."

*Final Word: If They Keep Ignoring, We'll Keep Shouting*

We're done being quiet. We're done sanitizing our stories so the world stays comfortable.

You're not dramatic. You're not "too much." You're surviving blood loss, paying the bills, raising kids, working jobs, and still showing up. That's power.

And if society keeps looking away? We'll hand them a microphone and a crime scene.

# 8

# Period Myths That Need to Die (Preferably in a Fire)

People will believe the Earth is flat before they'll believe the truth about periods—especially menorrhagia. Somehow menstrual blood is "dirty," cramps are "normal," and if you just drank enough kale smoothies your uterus would chill.

Nope. Not today.

Let's line these myths up and torch them.

*Myth #1: "It's Just a Heavy Period"*

That's like calling a bus crash "just a bump."

A regular period is drizzle. Menorrhagia is a monsoon. You're not spotting—you're flooding. You're not cramping—you're contracting.

*Myth #2: "You're Overreacting"*

Sweetheart, *I* didn't overreact—my uterus did. I was minding my business when it staged *Battle of the Bastards*.

Overreacting is crying over bangs gone wrong. Surviving monthly internal war crimes? That's called reality.

*Myth #3: "You Could Fix It with Better Self-Care"*

The wellness girls say: hydrate, eat chia, chant affirmations, align with the moon.

I've drunk pond-flavored smoothies, twisted into yoga pretzels, mooed on kale—and still bled like I was stabbed by a ghost.

You don't cure menorrhagia with vibes and oat milk.

*Myth #4: "It's Supposed to Hurt"*

Pain that makes you faint or scream into a pillow isn't "part of womanhood." It's a symptom of a condition society dismisses.

If your uterus feels like it's throwing Molotov cocktails, that's not normal—it's medical.

43

*Myth #5: "Periods Sync Because of Magic"*

No menstrual fairy, no lunar witchcraft. We're not syncing—we're just all oppressed at the same time.

And in one house? That's not sisterhood. That's mayhem. One bathroom. Two pads left. Good luck.

*Myth #6: "You Can't Get Pregnant on Your Period"*

Yes. You. Can.

Sperm hangs around for days. Irregular cycles mean surprises. So while you're bleeding like a crime scene, conception is still on the table. Wrap it up—even while you're wrapped in blankets.

*Myth #7: "You're Not Bleeding That Much"*

Really? Then explain why my pads look like crime exhibits and tampons can't last one Netflix episode.

For the record: over 80ml per cycle = menorrhagia. We triple that. This isn't bleeding. It's draining.

*Myth #8: "Tampons Take Your Virginity"*

Virginity isn't a body part, it's a social construct. Your hymen isn't a security tag.

If you can't handle cotton, how are you handling anything else?

*Myth #9: "Period Blood Is Dirty"*

So nosebleeds are fine, scraped knees are fine, but the blood that literally sustains humanity is "gross"?

Period blood isn't dirty. It's biology. It's life. And if you can watch zombies disemboweled on TV but can't handle a pad? That's your problem.

*Myth #10: "Menstrual Cups Work for Everyone"*

Great if your flow is polite. For the rest of us? That cup fills faster than a McDonald's soda. Remove it too slow and suddenly you're in a *Dexter* reboot.

They work for some, not for all. Stop treating them like gospel.

*Bonus Myth: "Bleeding Is a Gift"*

A yoga instructor once told me, *"Honor your sacred bleed."*

Sis, I just passed a jellyfish-sized clot and taste metal in my mouth. Nothing about this feels sacred. You know what would be sacred? Healthcare, paid leave, and free pads.

*Final Word*

Every myth fuels silence, shame, and suffering. So the next time someone repeats one? Smile, lean in close, and say:

*"Tell that to my ruined mattress, bitch."*

# 9

# Emergency Room or Just Another Tuesday?

Ever bled so much you thought, *"Should I go to the ER?"* ...but didn't, because it happens every month? Welcome to menorrhagia.

At this point, you develop a sixth sense. You don't panic. You don't scream. You just glance at a clot the size of a kiwi and think, *"Hmm. New one."* Flush. Wash hands. Back to your Zoom call.

For us, what should qualify as a medical emergency is just another Tuesday.

*What's "Normal"?*

The line between "period" and "problem" disappears fast. You bleed through a tampon and pad in 20 minutes. You're lightheaded. You pass clots that belong in a produce aisle. You should call someone—

but you don't.

Because the last time you went, you got a $900 bill and told to "monitor your flow." Monitor it? Sis, I'm hemorrhaging like a duel gone wrong.

*The ER Checklist*

Here's how it usually goes:

- Wrap a coat around your waist like you escaped a crime scene.
- Whisper "vaginal bleeding" to the receptionist while she shouts "WHAT KIND?"
- Fill out paperwork with hands shaking from cramps.
- Wait two hours on a tortilla-chip hospital pad.
- Finally get called back, pee in a cup, and answer the inevitable *"Could you be pregnant?"*
- Doctor breezes in, says, *"We don't see active hemorrhaging,"* and sends you home with iron and instructions to "follow up."

You leave broke, exhausted, and still bleeding.

*When Is It Actually Serious?*

That's the mindf***—you don't know anymore. Gaslit so many times, you no longer trust your instincts.

Is this fainting-level? ER-worthy? Or will they just shrug again while you bleed through a hospital chair?

If a man lost this much blood, they'd start a transfusion. You? *"Have you tried birth control?"*

*The Clot Horror Show*

Passing clots is traumatizing. They feel like organs sliding out. You sit, hear the *thwomp,* look down, panic, flush before you process it. Then you crawl back to bed praying you don't pass another.

Tell a doctor? *"That's common."*

Yeah, so is death. Doesn't mean I want to normalize it.

*The "Not Serious Enough" Olympics*

You: *"I'm bleeding too much."*
  Them: *"Not enough to intervene."*
  You: *"My cramps make me gasp."*
  Them: *"Unfortunate, but not life-threatening."*
  You: *"I'm passing clots the size of eggs."*

49

Them: *"Well, they're not blocking anything."*

Apparently you need to audition for *The Walking Dead* before they'll care.

## The "Wait and See" Death Sentence

Their favorite line: *"Let's wait and see."*

Wait for what? Fainting in Target? Passing out on a bus? Ending up on TikTok while EMTs drag you out of a Ross?

It's easy to "wait" when you're not the one soaking through chairs in public.

## The Bill on Top of the Blood Loss

The cherry on top: the invoice. Hundreds—sometimes thousands—for being told, *"You're fine."*

Ambulance? Don't even think about it. That's $1,200 to bleed in the back of a van. Better to Uber with a towel.

## DIY Triage

So you become your own medic. You assess:

- Pads per hour.
- Level of dizziness.
- Clot size versus fruit scale.

- Call GYN, mom, or 911?

Half the time, you just ride it out. Because you know the ER won't fix it—they'll just charge rent for ignoring you.

*Final Word: Bleeding Shouldn't Be a Gamble*

You shouldn't have to wonder if today's bloodbath is "ER-worthy" or just another ignored Tuesday. You shouldn't have to triage your own organs because the system can't be bothered.

So next time you ask, *"Should I go to the ER?"* also ask, *"Do I have the energy to be dismissed today?"*

If not, sit down, hydrate, curse the system, and add "ER roulette" to the list of games you never wanted to play. And the cruelest part? If men ever bled like this, you know damn well the system would've fixed it decades ago.

# 10

# If Men Bled Like This, We'd Have a Cure by Now

Let's just say it:

If men bled out of their d*cks every month-unpredictable, sheet-ruining, iron-sucking blood-baths, there would've been a cure before the moon landing.

You think they'd be handed jumbo pads and told to "tough it out"?

You think they'd accept iron pills and *"wait and see"*?

Hell no.

There would be press conferences. There would be Menstrual Freedom Day parades. Walgreens would have Flow Lounges with hot towels, snacks, and sports on TV.

*The Male Menstruation Tech Boom*

If it were them? The products would be wild:

- NASA-engineered tampons.
- Pads with Bluetooth and climate control.
- Period underwear with built-in speakers and Venmo.
- Government-funded menstrual leave with bonuses.
- Flow detectors in cars, chairs, and gaming consoles.

And all of it fully covered by insurance, advertised during the Super Bowl.

Meanwhile, we're still paying $12.99 for cotton tubes wrapped in shame.

*The Doctor Conversation, If It Were Them*

- Him: *"Doc, I'm bleeding out of my genitals."*
- Doctor: *"Sounds like stress. Drink water."*
- Him: *"It happens every month."*
- Doctor: *"Monitor it."*
- Him: *"I'm passing clots the size of golf balls."*
- Doctor: *"That's just part of being a man."*

Yeah right. He'd riot. Congress would declare a

national emergency. Mayo Clinic would open an entire Men's Flow Wing.

## The Praise Olympics

If men woke up in blood, they'd get medals.

"Bro, you came to work? Respect."

"Yeah, man, bled through my khakis on the way, but I'm here."

Standing ovation. Hero's discount at Chipotle.

Meanwhile, women call out sick and get side-eye from HR.

## The Menstrual Safety Act

If it were them, the workplace would change overnight.

Every bathroom stocked with pads, tampons, period-proof boxers, heating pads, and a snack bar. Blood-proof office chairs by law. "Flow Miles" on every airline. Telethons with Ryan Seacrest hosting *Stop the Bleed 2025*.

Instead? We get a sad dispenser with a 50¢ tampon from 1998.

*Meanwhile, Reality*

Men take a day off for a cold. Imagine them bleeding, cramping, fainting, and clotting for a week. They'd quit, sue, and demand reparations.

If periods hit men, the 40-hour week would be illegal. Women would be hailed as evolutionary gods for surviving it. Larry from accounting would be curled in the break room, whispering, *"Why didn't anyone warn me?!"*

*But Here We Are*

No medals. No leave. No praise.

Just us—bleeding through leggings, lying on heating pads, whispering *"I'm fine"* through gritted teeth. We're miracle workers, holding jobs and families together while scrubbing blood out of mattresses at 6 a.m.

And society still says, *"It's just a period."*

*Final Mic Drop*

The problem was never science. It was priorities.

Erectile dysfunction got billion-dollar pills. Menorrhagia got shame, silence, and a tampon tax.

But we're done suffering quietly.

We're bleeding loud—through aisles, ERs, workplaces, and these pages. And until society catches up? Consider this book the protest sign your uterus has been waving all along.

# 11

# The Last Word

If you made it this far, congratulations — you survived the Red Wedding in book form. You've laughed, you've cringed, you've nodded in painful solidarity. Maybe you even threw your heating pad at the wall once or twice.

Here's the truth: menorrhagia is not just a period problem. It's a life problem. It steals your sleep, your money, your patience, and sometimes your sanity. And yet, here you are — still working, still parenting, still showing up, still cracking jokes through the cramps.

That's not weakness. That's a superpower.

So the next time someone tries to minimize your pain, hand them this book. Let them read what it's like to wake up in a crime scene once a month and still go to work like nothing happened.

And if you've ever felt alone in this? You're not.

You've got an entire sisterhood out here bleeding through jeans, flipping mattresses, canceling plans, and still thriving.

This book isn't just a vent. It's a middle finger to shame, a roast of society's ignorance, and a reminder that you're tougher than you think.

We may not have a cure yet. We may not have national tampon subsidies. We may not even have doctors who believe us half the time.

But what we *do* have? Each other. Our voices. Our stories. Our rage. Our humor.

And that's enough to keep bleeding LOUD until somebody finally listens.

Mic dropped. Pads stacked. Uterus undefeated.

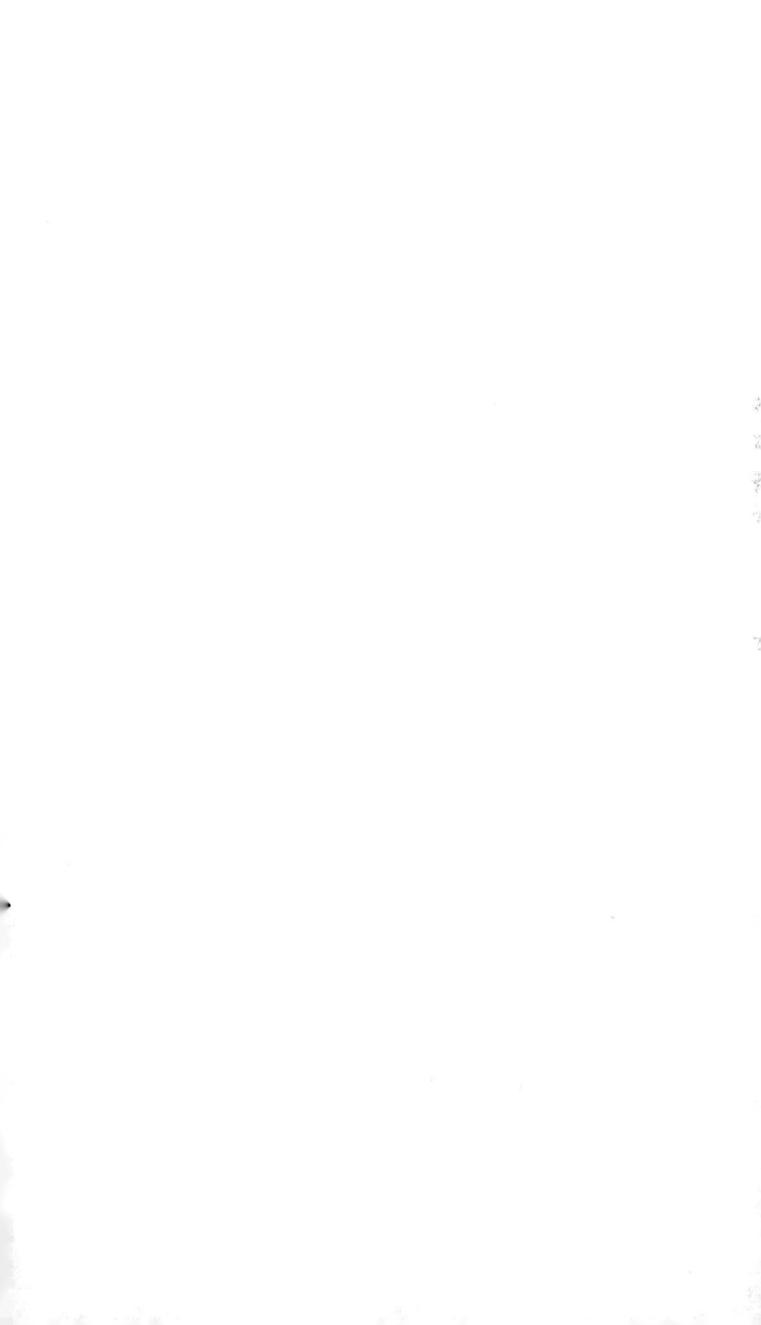

Printed in Dunstable, United Kingdom